COMPLETE DIARY FREE DIET RECIPES COOKBOOK

GEORGE ANDERSON

CHAPTER ONE

WHAT IS DAIRY?

Dairy

A dairy is a business enterprise established for the harvesting or processing (or both) of animal milk mostly from cows or buffaloes, but also from goats, sheep, horses, or camels for human consumption. A dairy is typically located on a dedicated dairy farm or in a section of a multi-purpose farm (mixed farm) that is concerned with the harvesting of milk.

As an attributive, the word dairy refers to milk-based products, derivatives and processes, and the animals and workers involved in their production: for example dairy cattle, dairy goat. A dairy farm produces milk and a dairy factory processes it into a variety of dairy products. These establishments constitute the global dairy industry, part of the food industry.

What is an intolerance?

Most often this refers to an intolerance to lactose, the sugar naturally found in milk (cow, goat and sheep). We make an enzyme in our intestine called lactase, which breaks down the lactose in milk allowing it to be absorbed. As we age, some of us fail to produce sufficient amounts of lactase and without it, the sugar ferments in the gut. An intolerance to dairy is less severe than an allergy but it may still lead to digestive, skin and inflammatory symptoms. However, if your intolerance isn't due to lactose, it's likely to be caused by the protein component of milk.

Those with an intolerance may find they're able to consume small amounts of milk with no ill-effects, particularly the products which have been processed such as live yogurt or cottage cheese. Some people find it easier to tolerate the milk of goat, sheep or buffalo, rather than cow's milk. We're all different and you'll need to establish your personal tolerance levels.

Who else might follow a dairy-free diet?

Some people prefer to avoid dairy for other reasons perhaps they dislike the taste, they have a cultural preference or because they feel better without it.

WHAT ARE THE HEALTH IMPLICATIONS OF A DAIRY-FREE DIET?

Milk is nutrient dense and makes a useful contribution towards our nutrient intake from providing a protein source to supplying minerals like calcium and iodine as well as vitamins such as the B group and vitamin A.

We typically value dairy foods for their calcium content but, fortunately, there are plenty of alternative food sources such as green leafy vegetables and nuts and fish with bones, such as tinned sardines. Speak to your GP if you suspect you may be at risk of a nutritional deficiency, including a calcium deficiency.

In the UK, milk and dairy products are also one of the main sources of iodine.

This little-talked-about nutrient is important for thyroid function. Those most at risk are young girls and pregnant women.

How will I know which foods to omit on a dairy-free diet?

Eating dairy-free involves omitting any product containing milk these include the obvious ones like butter, yogurt, cream and cheese but you will also need to check labels for the following:

- Casein/caseinates
- Whey
- Ghee (though vegetable ghee is fine)
- Buttermilk
- Hydrolysed casein/whey
- Lactalbumin
- Lactose

Don't forget milk and milk derivatives are likely to be found in:

• Batter (for pancakes, waffles, fish fingers etc.)

• Bread – many enriched breads will include butter and/or milk

• Low-fat and vegetable spreads

• Synthetic cream

• Crème pâtissière and custard

• Sweeteners

HOW SHOULD I GO ABOUT A DAIRY-FREE DIET?

• Audit your cupboards and food stores, and replace products containing dairy or dairy derivatives with suitable alternatives

• Get into the habit of reading labels

• Create a 'safe' list of the foods you enjoy and eat most often

• Be dairy savvy if a product is labelled 'dairy-free' – this only applies to cow's milk, not to other animal milks.

How to Start a Dairy-Free Diet

Dairy can play an important nutritional role in your diet because it's rich in nutrients like calcium, protein, and vitamins. But it's not the only source of those nutrients. Many people choose to follow a dairy-free diet because of an allergy or intolerance, personal preference, or ethical reasons.

While it may sound challenging to eliminate all dairy from your diet, with the right nutritional substitutions, going dairy-free can be a healthy, stress-free option.

WHAT IS A DAIRY-FREE DIET?

Simply put, a dairy-free diet excludes all (or most) dairy products. This includes milk from any animal in addition to foods and drinks that contain milk, such as cheese, yogurt, butter, and cream.

Are Vegan and Dairy-Free the Same Thing?

You might be wondering, is a vegan diet a dairy-free diet? Though they do have similarities, they're not quite the same.

• A vegan diet eliminates any product that's made from an animal. This includes dairy, meat, eggs, and fish.

• A dairy-free diet excludes all or most dairy products. This includes milk and any foods made with milk.

One way to think of it is that while all vegan food is dairy-free, not all dairy-free food is vegan.

BENEFITS AND RISKS

As with any diet, there are benefits and potential risks to going dairy-free. This is because deleting a food group subsequently removes calories and nutrients from your diet.

The benefits and risks of a dairy-free diet can vary depending on the person, their understanding of a balanced diet, their current dietary patterns, and their individual needs.

Benefits and Advantages

One benefit to a dairy-free diet is that it is considered generally safe to follow indefinitely as long as nutritional needs are met.

In addition, a dairy-free diet is beneficial for those who have:

• Lactose intolerance (trouble digesting the sugar in milk)

• Cow's milk allergy

• Other sensitivity to dairy products

Relief from uncomfortable symptoms like bloating, gas, abdominal pain, and diarrhea can resolve within a few days after you stop eating dairy products.

Risks and Disadvantages

One concern with going dairy-free is making sure you get enough of the nutrients your body needs to function properly. Dairy can be a major source of calcium and vitamin D, and deficiencies in those nutrients can potentially lead to bone density issues.

Another disadvantage worth mentioning is that many milk substitutes and other dairy-free items are significantly more expensive than their dairy counterparts and are not found in all grocery stores across the country. The cost and availability factors make going without dairy less accessible to people living in historically marginalized communities, contributing to barriers to heathy eating and health equity.

Lastly, making a major change to your diet like strictly avoiding dairy can be challenging and will require some planning ahead on grocery shopping and cooking.

Pros and Cons

Advantages to going dairy-free:

• Generally safe and can be followed as long as nutritional needs are met

• Helps ease discomfort of lactose intolerance or dairy allergy

• May potentially help contribute to weight loss

Drawbacks to going dairy-free:

• Not getting enough nutrients

• Alternate foods may be costly or inaccessible

• Strictly avoiding dairy can be difficult, and requires planning to meet nutritional needs

FOODS TO EAT VS. FOODS TO AVOID

Figuring out what you should and should not eat on a dairy-free diet is a first step to getting started.

In general, you'll want to look for and eat:

• Milk substitutes

• Dairy-free foods rich in calcium, protein, and vitamin D

• Products labeled "dairy-free" and "nondairy" (with caution)

In general, you'll want to avoid:

• Cow's milk and other animal milks

- Foods made from milk (such as cheese, yogurt, and ice cream)

- Foods that contain or are prepared with milk (such as baked goods and salad dressings)

- Foods that may come into contact with milk (such as some deli meats and dark chocolate)

How to Read Food Labels

By law, food products containing any of the nine major food allergens are required to have plain-language labels (such as "contains dairy") to help people avoid them. Milk is one of those allergens, but it's still a good idea to read the label and ingredients list carefully.

- Products labeled "dairy-free": The Food and Drug Administration (FDA) doesn't regulate this term, so these products could still contain casein milk derivatives like casein (a milk protein) or whey.

• Products labeled "nondairy": FDA regulations technically allow these products to contain a very small percentage of milk by weight in the form of casein.

Dairy-Free Nutrition

While the Department of Agriculture (USDA) recommends low-fat dairy products as part of a balanced diet, it acknowledges that there are other ways to meet your nutritional needs if you can't or prefer not to consume dairy.

The nutrients found in dairy foods like calcium and vitamin D help support bone health and immune function, so you'll want to make sure you get enough of those nutrients from another source.

Further, if you cut dairy from your diet for health or potential weight loss reasons, you'll want to make sure you're still consuming enough calories each day to keep your body functioning properly.

MEAL PLANNING WHEN DAIRY-FREE

Following a dairy-free diet usually requires some planning, but the guidelines are simpler than you might think.

To help build a healthy meal plan, first focus on getting in three to five servings of fruit and vegetables in per day. From there, you have several options for dairy-free alternatives:

• Milk substitutes: Alternatives like soy, almond, coconut, and oat milk can replace cow's milk. Just be aware that their nutritional content can vary greatly.

• Protein: While dairy is a good source of protein, you can often get your fill of it from lean meats. If you are avoiding animal products, you can also get protein from plant-based options and other products like beans, lentils, legumes, nuts, seeds, soy milk, and eggs.

• Calcium: Consider foods that have been fortified with calcium, such as orange juice and cereals, or foods naturally high in calcium, such as kale, tofu, chia seeds, and almond butter.

• Vitamin D: In addition to (safe) sunlight exposure, solid nondairy dietary sources of vitamin D include eggs, fatty fish, and fortified cereals.

• Riboflavin (vitamin B2): Leafy greens, sweet potatoes, whole grains, and meat can be good sources for this essential vitamin.

• Phosphorus: This nutrient can be found in meat, fatty fish, legumes, or bread.

THE BENEFITS OF EATING DAIRY FREE

Embracing A Lifestyle Change

Embarking on a dairy free lifestyle may be daunting at first, especially if it's due to a recently diagnosed milk intolerance or allergy. While health fiends and dieticians have raved about the benefits of going dairy free for years, it's much more difficult to convert when milk, cheese and butter are a big part of your diet... Not to mention the occasional dairy laden dessert! Many also still think that avoiding dairy makes your meals less tasty, filling and nutritious, but this just isn't the case.

If you're converting to a dairy free diet with an intolerance or allergy, or if you're simply making the switch out of choice, we can make the transition that bit easier. Helping you to move from Dairy Queen to Team Dairy Free with confidence and positivity, we've summarised the key benefits of cutting out the milk.

Drop The Pounds

One of the top benefits of cutting out dairy is the removal of excess saturated fats, sugar and salt from your diet, thus lessening your calorie intake and promoting a healthy weight. Dairy is also renowned as an acidic food, disrupting your body's acid/alkaline balance. When you remove it from your diet, digestion becomes much more effective and helps to shift those pesky extra pounds.

Say Bye To The Bloat

When you switch to a dairy free diet, one of the first benefits you'll notice is a flatter stomach. If you're prone to bloating then cutting out milk products can make a significant difference. This is because your gut can't tolerate dairy as well as other foods, leading to swelling and discomfort. Dairy is also linked to constipation, so swapping it for more fibrous alternatives makes it easier to 'go'.

Heighten Your Senses

Many dairy free converts have discovered the added bonus of a better sense of smell. Casein, the protein in dairy, is closely linked to excessive mucus production, which in turn leads to a blocked nose and sinus pressure. Saying no to dairy can help to reduce this congestion and banish your runny nose. Our tastebuds also change depending on the food we consume, so cutting out the overpowering flavours of dairy means you'll appreciate other tastes more.

Get That Glow

The dairy free lifestyle is renowned for its benefits on the skin, particularly for those that suffer from conditions like dryness, eczema and psoriasis. Turning down the milk helps to clear your skin, banish those dry and itchy patches, and provide a bright, youthful glow. The dairy free diet has also been found to help those suffering with acne, though the results are dependent on your individual dermatological condition.

Try New Things

The dairy free diet provides you with a great opportunity to try new food. Prior to your switch, you probably would have never considered creamy cashew nut yoghurt , sweet coconut milk ice cream or an indulgent almond milk rice pudding. Now, it's time to expand your palate and experiment with new recipes! Dairy free also sees an increase in focus on fruit, veg, nuts and pulses, which are all very nutritious and beneficial to the body. And don't worry, you can still ensure you're consuming enough calcium by eating almonds and green vegetables.

The benefits of removing dairy from your diet are plentiful, improving your physical health as well as refreshing your mind. And what's more, dairy free alternatives can be whipped up into delicious recipes that are more nutritious for your body and kinder to your waistline. Why not see the results for yourself?

Refresh And Revitalise

Switching to dairy free food can see your energy levels soar, with many claiming they've never felt so great. This is because milk products are naturally high in the amino acid tryptophan, which promotes tiredness. Dairy is also harder to digest than other food, causing your body to use more energy. When you cut back, you'll notice an increase in energy and focus, contributing to your overall sense of wellbeing.

CHAPTER TWO

DAIRY FREE DIET RECIPES

Here are some dairy free recipes one can try if jumping on the dairy diet, each one of the recipes are explained by listing the ingredients alongside the instructions on how to go about it;

Many-Veggie Vegetable Soup

Ingredients

- 2 tablespoons extra-virgin olive oil
- 1 medium yellow onion, diced
- Sea salt and fresh black pepper
- 1 medium carrot, diced
- 1 small sweet potato, diced
- ¼ cup dry white wine, i.e., pinot grigio

- 1 14.5-ounce can diced fire roasted tomatoes

- 4 garlic cloves, chopped

- 2 teaspoons dried oregano, or 2 tablespoons chopped fresh thyme or rosemary

- ¼ teaspoon red pepper flakes, more to taste

- 4 cups vegetable broth

- 2 bay leaves

- 1 cup halved cherry tomatoes

- 1 cup chopped green beans

- 1 zucchini, diced

- 1 15-ounce can chickpeas, drained and rinsed

- 2 tablespoons white wine vinegar

- 1½ cups chopped kale

Instructions

1. Heat the oil in a large pot over medium heat. Add the onion, ½ teaspoon salt, and several grinds of pepper, and cook, stirring occasionally, for 8 minutes. Add the carrot and sweet potato, stir and cook 2 more minutes.

2. Add the wine and cook for about 30 seconds to reduce by half, then add the canned tomatoes, garlic, oregano, and red pepper flakes. Stir in the broth and bay leaves. Bring to a boil, then reduce the heat to a simmer and cook, covered, for 20 minutes.

3. Stir in the cherry tomatoes, green beans, zucchini, chickpeas, and cover and cook 10 to 15 more minutes, until the green beans are tender.

4. Stir in the vinegar, kale, an additional ½ teaspoon salt (or to taste), and more pepper.

Yakisoba Chicken

INGREDIENTS

- 1/2 teaspoon sesame oil

- 1 tablespoon canola oil

- 2 tablespoons chili paste

- cloves garlic, chopped

- 4 skinless, boneless chicken breast halves, sliced into 1-inch cubes

- 1/2 cup soy sauce, divided

- 1 onion, sliced lengthwise into eights

- 1/2 medium head cabbage, chopped

- 2 carrots, chopped

- 8 ounces soba noodles, cooked and drained

DIRECTIONS

• In a large skillet, pour the sesame oil, canola oil, and chili paste. Stir for 30 seconds on medium heat.

• Add the garlic and stir for 30 seconds. Cook the chicken with 1/4 cup of soy sauce for 5 minutes, or until no longer pink. Remove from the pan and set aside.

• Add the onion, cabbage, and carrots to the same skillet. Fry for 2 to 3 minutes, or until the cabbage starts to wilt.

• Increase the heat to high and mix in the remaining soy sauce, cooked noodles, and chicken mixture for 1 minute or until combined. Serve and enjoy!

Vegan Spinach Salad with Maple Balsamic Dressing

INGREDIENTS

Spinach Salad Base

- 6 cups spinach

- ½ cup pecans

- ½ cup dry cranberries

- ¾ cup cucumber

- 1 medium avocado

- ¼ cup hemp seeds

- ½ cup green onion

Balsamic Dressing

- 3 tablespoons balsamic vinegar

- 1 tablespoon Dijon mustard

- 2 tablespoons maple syrup

- 2 tablespoons extra virgin olive oil

* ½ teaspoon salt

INSTRUCTIONS

1. Prepare salad ingredients by chopping them and adding to a salad bowl. 6 cups spinach,½ cup pecans,½ cup dry cranberries,¾ cup cucumber,1 medium avocado,¼ cup hemp seeds,½ cup green onion

2. Whisk together the dressing ingredients or shake together in a jar. 3 tablespoons balsamic vinegar,1 tablespoon Dijon mustard,2 tablespoons maple syrup,2 tablespoons extra virgin olive oil,½ teaspoon salt

3. Toss the salad with dressing before serving and enjoy!

Coca Cola Pulled Pork

INGREDIENTS

- 4 to 5 pounds of pork roast (shoulder or butt)

- 2 teaspoons garlic, minced and dehydrated

- 2 teaspoons onion, minced, dehydrated

- 1/4 teaspoon black pepper, ground

- 1/4 teaspoon cayenne pepper, ground

- 1 teaspoon liquid smoke

- 1 liter Coca-Cola (or other cola brands)

- 20 ounces barbecue sauce

DIRECTIONS

- Place pork roast in a 5-quart Crockpot. Season the pork with garlic, onion, and black and cayenne peppers. Pour in the liquid smoke and Coke until they cover the roast.

• Set the Crockpot to low heat and cook for 8 to 10 hours.

• Transfer the roast into a serving platter. Discard the bones and trim the fat. Shred the pork into thin strands with 2 forks. Coat with barbecue sauce. Serve and enjoy!

Best Roasted Vegetables (Perfectly Seasoned!)

Ingredients

• 1 medium head cauliflower (2 pounds)

• 1 crown broccoli (1/2 pound)

• 1 medium red onion

• 2 medium sweet potatoes (1 1/2 pounds)

- 1 red pepper

- 1 yellow pepper

- 4 tablespoons olive oil

- 2 teaspoons garlic powder

- 2 teaspoons Old Bay seasoning

- 1 teaspoon kosher salt

Instructions

1. Adjust the oven racks for roasting 2 trays. Preheat the oven to 450 degrees Fahrenheit.

2. Chop the vegetables: Chop the cauliflower and broccoli into florets. Chop the onion into 1/2-inch slices. Cut the sweet potato in half lengthwise, in half again lengthwise, and then cut each quarter into thin pie-shaped slices (see the photo). Chop the peppers into 1/2-inch strips, then cut the strips in half.

3. Line two baking sheets with parchment paper (we prefer this to silicone baking mats because it results in crispier veggies). Spread the vegetables evenly onto each sheet. Drizzle half the olive oil onto each tray, then with half the seasonings onto each tray. Mix with your hands until evenly coated.

4. Place into the oven and bake for 20 minutes (do not stir!). Remove the pans from the oven, rotate them, and roast another 10 minutes (for 30 minutes total) until tender and lightly browned on one side. Transfer to a serving bowl or dish and serve immediately.

Coca Cola Chicken

INGREDIENTS

• 4 skinless, boneless chicken breast halves

• Salt and pepper, to taste

• 2 tablespoons Worcestershire sauce

• 1 cup ketchup

• 1 cup Coca-Cola or any cola-flavored carbonated drink

DIRECTIONS

• Preheat the oven to 350 degrees Fahrenheit.

• In a 9×13-inch baking dish, layer the chicken in a single layer. Season with salt and pepper.

• In a medium bowl, stir together Worcestershire sauce, ketchup, and Coke until well combined. Pour the mixture over the chicken. Cover the dish with aluminum foil.

• Bake for 50 minutes or until the chicken is no longer pink. Use a meat thermometer to ensure doneness. Cooked chicken has an internal temperature of 165 degrees Fahrenheit. Enjoy!

Sweet Potato Salad Recipe

Ingredients

• 4 medium sweet potatoes, peeled and chopped (2 lb before peeling)

• 1 onion, diced

• 1/2 tsp salt, and optional pepper

• 3 tbsp oil, or spray (for fat-free option)

• 2 tsp minced garlic

• 2 tbsp lime juice

- 1 red bell pepper, diced

- 1 can black beans, or 1 1/2 cups cooked

- optional 1 cup canned or cooked corn

- 3/4 cup fresh cilantro, chopped (omit if desired)

Instructions

- Toss sweet potatoes and onions with 1 1/2 tbsp oil (or spray) and the garlic, sprinkle with salt and optional pepper, and arrange in a single layer on two parchment-lined baking sheets. Place in a non-preheated oven on the center rack, then turn the oven to 450 F. Bake 35 minutes, or until potatoes are soft. Add all remaining ingredients to a large bowl, then toss with the sweet potatoes. Serve hot or cold.

Trisha Yearwood Sloppy Joes

INGREDIENTS

- 3 tablespoons olive oil

- 1 medium onion, finely diced

- 1 medium bell pepper, finely diced

- 1 pound ground beef

- One 15-ounce can diced fire-roasted tomatoes

- One 15-ounce can kidney beans, drained and rinsed

- 1/4 cup tomato paste

- 2 tablespoons apple cider vinegar

- 1 teaspoon brown sugar

- Kosher salt and freshly ground black pepper

- 4 hamburger buns

DIRECTIONS

- In a large skillet, start the olive oil over medium heat.

- Toss in the bell peppers and onions, then cook until tender, maybe 10 minutes.

- Place the ground beef in the skillet and cook until browned, breaking it up with a spatula as you go.

- Mix in the beans, tomatoes, brown sugar, vinegar, and tomato paste.

- Add salt and pepper to taste, and simmer for 10 to 15 minutes.

- Place generous scoops of meat on the warmed hamburger buns.

Zesty Lime Shrimp And Avocado Salad

INGREDIENTS

- 1/4 cup chopped red onion

- 2 limes, juice of

- 1 tsp olive oil

- 1/4 tsp kosher salt, black pepper to taste

- 1 lb jumbo cooked, peeled shrimp, chopped*

- 1 medium tomato, diced

- 1 medium hass avocado, diced (about 5 oz)

- 1 jalapeno, seeds removed, diced fine

- 1 tbsp chopped cilantro

INSTRUCTIONS

1. In a small bowl combine red onion, lime juice, olive oil, salt and pepper. Let them marinate at least 5 minutes to mellow the flavor of the onion.

2. In a large bowl combine chopped shrimp, avocado, tomato, jalapeño.

3. Combine all the ingredients together, add cilantro and gently toss. Adjust salt and pepper to taste.

Best Vegan Pizza

Ingredients

- 1 small head broccoli, florets chopped into small pieces, top of stalk diced (½ cup)

- ⅓ cup halved cherry tomatoes

- kernels from 1 ear fresh corn

- ¼ cup coarsely chopped red onion

- ½ jalapeño, thinly sliced

- 4 oil-packed sun-dried tomatoes, diced

- extra-virgin olive oil, for drizzling and brushing

- 1 (16-ounce) ball of pizza dough

- ½ cup fresh basil leaves

- 2 tablespoons fresh thyme leaves

- pinches of red pepper flakes

- sea salt and freshly ground black pepper

- Cashew Cream

Instructions

1. Preheat the oven to 450°F.

2. In a medium bowl, combine the broccoli, tomatoes, corn, onion, jalapeño, and sun-dried tomatoes and drizzle with olive oil and pinches of salt and pepper. Toss to coat and taste. The vegetables should be well-seasoned and well-coated with the olive oil so that the vegetables are flavorful throughout the pizza.

3. Stretch the pizza dough onto a 14-inch pizza pan. Brush the outer edges of

the dough lightly with olive oil and spoon a few scoops of cashew cream onto the center of the dough, just enough to spread it into a thin layer. Distribute the vegetables onto the dough.

4. Bake 15 minutes, or until the crust is golden, cooked through, and the broccoli is tender and roasted. Remove from the oven and drizzle generously with the cashew cream (if your cashew cream is too thick to drizzle, stir in a little water). Top with the fresh basil, fresh thyme, and pinches of red pepper flakes.

Trisha Yearwood's Meatloaf Recipe

INGREDIENTS

- 2 pounds lean ground beef

- 20 saltine crackers, crushed into crumbs

- 1 large egg, slightly beaten

- 1/2 cup ketchup

- 1 tablespoon mustard

- 1 teaspoon salt

- 1/2 teaspoon pepper

- 1/2 yellow onion, finely chopped

- Optional: white bread slices, lettuce, and tomato for sandwiches

DIRECTIONS

- Preheat the oven to 350 degrees Fahrenheit.

- Combine the beef, cracker crumbs, egg, ketchup, mustard, salt, pepper, and onion in a large bowl. Blend in a stand mixer just until combined.

- Form the mixture into two loaves and place them in a 9x3x2-inch baking pan, crosswise.

• Bake the loaves for an hour or until brown.

• Transfer the loaves into serving plates right away. Let them cool slightly to firm up.

• Slice, serve, and enjoy!

• *If making a sandwich, cut 2 slices of meatloaf. Place them on top of a slice of white bread, and top with lettuce and tomato. Cover with another piece of white bread.

Colorful Beet Salad with Carrot, Quinoa & Spinach

INGREDIENTS

Salad

• ½ cup uncooked quinoa, rinsed

• 1 cup frozen organic edamame

- ⅓ cup slivered almonds or pepitas (green pumpkin seeds)

- 1 medium raw beet, peeled

- 1 medium-to-large carrot (or 1 additional medium beet), peeled

- 2 cups packed baby spinach or arugula, roughly chopped

- 1 avocado, cubed

Vinaigrette

- 3 tablespoons apple cider vinegar

- 2 tablespoons lime juice

- 2 tablespoons olive oil

- 1 tablespoon chopped fresh mint or cilantro

- 2 tablespoons honey or maple syrup or agave nectar

- ½ to 1 teaspoon Dijon mustard, to taste

- ¼ teaspoon salt

- Freshly ground black pepper, to taste

INSTRUCTIONS

1. To cook the quinoa: First, rinse the quinoa in a fine mesh colander under running water for a minute or two. In a medium-sized pot, combine the rinsed quinoa and 1 cup water. Bring the mixture to a gentle boil, then cover the pot, reduce heat to a simmer and cook for 15 minutes. Remove the quinoa from heat and let it rest, still covered, for 5 minutes. Uncover the pot, drain off any excess water and fluff the quinoa with a fork. Set it aside to cool.

2. To cook the edamame: Bring a pot of water to boil, then add the frozen

edamame and cook just until the beans are warmed through, about 5 minutes. Drain and set aside.

3. To toast the almonds or pepitas: In a small skillet over medium heat, toast the almonds or pepitas, stirring frequently, until they are fragrant and starting to turn golden on the edges, about 5 minutes. Transfer to a large serving bowl to cool.

4. To prepare the beet(s) and/or carrot: First of all, feel free to just chop them as finely as possible using a sharp chef's knife OR grate them on a box grater. If you have a spiralizer, you can spiralize them using blade C, then chop the ribbons into small pieces using a sharp chef's knife. If you have a mandoline and julienne peeler (this is a pain), use the mandoline to julienne the beet and use a

julienne peeler to julienne the carrot, then chop the ribbons into small pieces using a sharp chef's knife.

5. To prepare the vinaigrette: Whisk together all of the ingredients until emulsified.

6. To assemble the salad: In your large serving bowl, combine the toasted almonds/pepitas, cooked edamame, prepared beet(s) and/or carrot, roughly chopped spinach/arugula (see note above about leftovers), cubed avocado and cooked quinoa.

7. Finally, drizzle dressing over the mixture (you might not need all of it) and gently toss to combine. You'll end up with a pink salad if you toss it really well! Season to taste with salt (up to an additional ¼ teaspoon) and black pepper. Serve.

Beef and Broccoli

INGREDIENTS

- 1/3 cup oyster sauce

- 2 teaspoons toasted sesame oil

- 1/3 cup sherry

- 1 teaspoon soy sauce

- 1 teaspoon granulated sugar

- 1 teaspoon cornstarch

- 3/4 pound beef flank steak, sliced into 1/8-inch thick cuts

- 3 tablespoons vegetable oil, more if needed

- 1 thin slice of fresh ginger root

- 1 clove garlic, peeled and smashed

- 1 pound broccoli, sliced into florets

DIRECTIONS

- In a bowl, combine oyster sauce, sesame oil, sherry, soy sauce, sugar, and cornstarch until sugar and cornstarch are dissolved.

- Place steak pieces in a large, shallow bowl. Pour over the oyster sauce mixture and coat steak pieces completely. Refrigerate to marinate for at least 30 minutes.

- Add vegetable oil in a large skillet or wok over medium-high heat. Add ginger and garlic and stir. Allow them to sizzle in the hot oil to flavor it, about 1 minute. Remove and discard ginger and garlic.

- Add the broccoli and stir until vibrant green and slightly tender, about 5 to 7 minutes. Take the broccoli out and set it aside.

- Add more oil into the wok if needed. Add the beef and marinade. Stir until the meat has browned, and the sauce is reduced into a glaze, about 5 minutes.

• Add the cooked broccoli. Stir meat and broccoli until heated through, about 3 minutes.

Creamy Salmon Pasta Recipe

Ingredients

- ☐8 oz. pasta (of choice)

- ☐4 salmon filets (skinless)

- ☐1/2 cup olive oil

- ☐1/2 cup almond flour

- ☐1 1/2 cups unsweetened almond milk

- ☐2 tsp garlic powder

- ☐salt/pepper (to taste)

Instructions

1. Cook the pasta according to directions, drain, and set aside.

2. Season the salmon filets with salt and pepper and set aside.

3. Cook the salmon filets with 1 Tbsp of the oil over medium heat for about 4-6 minutes on each side (or until it feels firm to the touch and is fully cooked).

4. While the salmon is cooking, whisk together the almond milk, garlic powder, and salt/pepper (to taste) in a mixing bowl until smooth.

5. Heat the olive oil in a sauce pan over medium-high heat.

6. Add in the almond flour and whisk to create a paste.

7. Add in the almond milk mixture and whisk, bringing to a simmer.

8. Continue to simmer and whisk continously for about 7-10 minutes as the sauce heats up, reduces, and thickens.

9. Remove from heat and let the sauce sit for about 3 minutes.

10. Add in the pasta and stir, coating it evenly in the creamy sauce.

11. Cut the salmon into small pieces and lightly mix it into the pasta and sauce.

12. Serve and enjoy!

Old-Fashioned Beef Stew

INGREDIENTS

- 2 pounds cubed beef stew meat

- 3 tablespoons vegetable oil

- 4 cubes beef bouillon, crumbled

- 4 cups of water

- 1 teaspoon dried rosemary

- 1 teaspoon dried parsley

- 1/2 teaspoon ground black pepper

- 3 large potatoes, peeled and cubed

- 4 carrots, cut into 1-inch pieces

- 4 stalks celery, cut into 1-inch pieces

- 1 large onion, chopped

- 2 teaspoons cornstarch

- 2 teaspoons cold water

DIRECTIONS

- Add the oil to a Dutch Oven, or a large, heavy-bottom pot.

- Cook the beef in batches over medium heat until brown. Ensure to cook on all sides and move to a plate while cooking the rest. Be careful not to overcrowd the pot.

• When the beef is all browned, dissolve the beef bouillon in hot water and then add to the pot.

• Carefully place the beef back into the pot, with the liquid and seasonings.

• Bring everything to a boil before reducing the heat to a low simmer and covering with the lid.

• Leave the beef to simmer for an hour, checking occasionally and stirring to prevent anything from sticking.

• While the beef cooks, wash, peel, and cut your vegetables. Be careful not to cut them too small, so that they keep their form after cooking.

• In a small bowl, make a u201cslurryu201d using the cornstarch and 2 teaspoons of water. Mix it thoroughly until totally smooth.

• After an hour, add in the vegetables and slurry, stirring everything through.

• Cover the pot and let simmer for another hour, stirring occasionally.

• Serve in a big bowl with crusty French bread.

BBQ Baked Beans

INGREDIENTS

• 1 pound ground beef

• 1 small onion, minced

• 2 tablespoons dry mesquite flavored seasoning mix

• (2) 28-ounce canned baked beans (such as Bush's Original)

- 1/4 cup molasses

- 3/4 cup brown sugar

- 3/4 cup barbeque sauce

- 2 teaspoons dry mustard powder

- 2 pinches cayenne pepper, or to taste

DIRECTIONS

- Preheat your oven to 350 degrees Fahrenheit.

- Place the ground beef, onion, and mesquite seasoning in a large skillet over medium heat. Keep stirring for 10 minutes, or until the beef has browned and broken up into crumbles.

- Transfer the mixture into a large baking dish, draining the excess liquid. Mix in the baked beans, molasses, brown sugar, barbeque sauce, dry mustard powder, and cayenne pepper. Mix until the sugar is dissolved.

• Bake the dish for 20 minutes, or until the beans start to bubble.

Mexican Buddha Bowl

INGREDIENTS

• 1 cup cooked brown rice (or quinoa)

• 1 cup black beans (drained and rinsed)

• 2 1/2 cups cherry tomatoes (halved)

• 1 avocado 1 cup corn

• Dressing: guacamole (optional)

• lime juice (optional)

• hummus (optional)

DIRECTIONS

• Cook the rice according to package instructions.

• While the rice is cooking, prepare the beans. For canned beans, first drain the liquid and rinse the beans. Place the beans in a saucepan and add enough water just to cover the beans.

• Cook the beans over medium heat. Bring to a boil and then cook for about 5 minutes. Set to the side. If you're using a 16oz can of beans, you'll be using half the can for this recipe.

• Prepare the corn. If you're using frozen corn, simply place it in the microwave and cook per package instructions.

• Combine all of your ingredients into a bowl. Combine the brown rice, black beans, cherry tomatoes, sliced avocado, and corn into a big round bowl.

• Top it off with your favorite dressing. A few tablespoons of guacamole, lime juice, or hummus.

• Enjoy!

Dreamy Vegan Cauliflower Alfredo Sauce

INGREDIENTS

• 1 teaspoon olive oil

• ½ yellow onion, chopped

• 3 cloves garlic, crushed

• 3 cups (12 ounces) chopped cauliflower

• 1 cup vegetable stock or water

• 1-2 tablespoons nutritional yeast, see notes

• 2 teaspoons lemon juice

• 1-2 teaspoons sea salt

• ½ teaspoon soy sauce, gluten-free or coco aminos, as needed

• Optional: 1 tablespoon butter, vegan or regular butter both work, use what you have on hand

INSTRUCTIONS

• Heat the oil in a medium-sized pot over medium-high heat. Add the onion and let it cook for 3-4 minutes, or until it is soft and translucent. Add the garlic and cook for 30 seconds. Add the cauliflower and the vegetable stock or water to the pot, cover with a lid and let the cauliflower steam for 5 minutes, or until it is soft.

1 teaspoon olive oil,½ yellow onion,3 cloves garlic,3 cups (12 ounces) chopped cauliflower,1 cup vegetable stock or water

• Transfer everything in the pot to a blender (a high-powered blender will make the smoothest sauce, but any blender will work) and blend on high until smooth. Add the remaining ingredients (starting with 1 tablespoon of nutritional yeast and 1 teaspoon of sea salt) and blend again. Taste and add more nutritional yeast and sea salt, if you'd like. If you are using the optional butter add it now and blend once more.

1-2 tablespoons nutritional yeast,2 teaspoons lemon juice,1-2 teaspoons sea salt,½ teaspoon soy sauce,Optional: 1 tablespoon butter

• Either use the cauliflower alfredo right away or pour it into a pan to keep warm until you are ready to use it.

15 Bean Soup (Easy Recipe)

INGREDIENTS

• 1 (1-pound) bag of regular 15 Bean Soup mix or Cajun 15 Bean Soup mix

• 2 tablespoons olive oil

- 2 to 3 ham hocks or 1 ham bone (meat included)

- 1 large onion, chopped

- 3 stalks celery (leaves included), chopped

- 4 garlic cloves, minced

- 1 (15 to 30-ounce) can whole tomatoes, crushed

- 1 tablespoon dried parsley

- 1 teaspoon dried rosemary

- 1 teaspoon salt

- 1 teaspoon ground black pepper

- 2 chicken bouillon cubes

DIRECTIONS

- Rinse the beans. Place them in a large pot and cover with water over medium-high heat. Bring the beans to a boil, stirring occasionally.

- Remove the pot from the heat and cover with a lid. Let the beans sit for an hour, then drain and set aside.

- Pour the olive oil into the pot over medium heat. Saute the ham hocks, onion, and celery until tender. Add the garlic and saute for 2 more minutes.

- Add the beans. Pour water until it's 2 inches above the beans.

- Stir in the tomatoes (juice included), parsley, rosemary, salt, pepper, and bouillon cubes.

- Bring the mixture to a boil, stirring occasionally. Reduce the heat to medium-low and cover the pot. Let it simmer, stirring occasionally, for 2 to 2 ½ hours or until the beans are tender.

Add more water if the mixture is getting too thick.

Creamy Butternut Squash Pasta

Ingredients

- ½ small butternut squash, halved vertically, and seeded

- Extra-virgin olive oil

- 2 shallots, coarsely chopped (½ cup)

- 3 garlic cloves, unpeeled

- ¾ cup water

- ½ cup raw cashews

- 1 tablespoon nutritional yeast

- 1 tablespoon balsamic vinegar

- 10 fresh sage leaves

- 1 tablespoon fresh thyme, plus a few leaves for garnish

- 12 ounces rotini pasta

- Sea salt and freshly ground black pepper

- Sauteed broccoli, for serving, optional

Instructions

1. Preheat the oven to 425°F and line a baking sheet with parchment paper.

2. Drizzle the squash with olive oil, sprinkle with salt and pepper, and place cut-side down on the baking sheet. Wrap the shallot and garlic cloves in foil with a drizzle of olive oil and a pinch of salt and place on the baking sheet. Roast for 30 minutes or until the squash is soft.

3. Scoop 1 cup of the squash flesh and transfer to a blender with the shallot, peeled garlic, water, cashews, 2 tablespoons olive oil, nutritional yeast, vinegar, sage, thyme, ¾ teaspoon salt,

and several grinds of black pepper. Blend until creamy.

4. Cook the pasta according to package directions in a pot of salted boiling water. Reserve 1 cup of the hot pasta water.

5. Drain the pasta and return to the pot. Stir in the sauce, adding 1/2 to 1 cup of the reserved pasta water to loosen the sauce and coat the pasta. Season with ¼ to ½ teaspoon salt. Top with freshly ground black pepper, a few thyme leaves and sautéed broccoli, if desired.

Chipotle Black Bean Soup Recipe

INGREDIENTS

- 2 tablespoons olive oil

- 1 yellow onion (finely diced)

- 4 cloves garlic (minced)

- 1 pound dried black beans (rinsed)

- 2 bay leaves

- 1 tsp cumin

- 1 tsp dried parsley

- 1 tsp dried oregano

- 1 tsp paprika

- 1/4 tsp chili powder (or to taste)

- 6 cups water (or more as needed)

- Juice of 1 lime

- Salt to taste

DIRECTIONS

- Rinse the beans thoroughly and remove any bad seeds from the bunch.

- Drizzle the olive oil into a large Dutch oven or stock pot over medium heat. Allow oil to warm up.

- Add the diced onion and cook for 3 to 5 minutes, or until softened.

- Add garlic and cook for about 30 seconds, or until fragrant.

- Stir in the black beans, dried parsley, oregano, cumin, and bay leaves. Add enough water to cover the beans.

- Bring to a boil and reduce heat to medium-low. Simmer for 2 hours or until beans are tender.

- Remove from heat and take out the bay leaves.

- Lastly, mix in the paprika, chili powder and lime juice. Season with salt. Squeeze some lemon or lime juice for a tangy twist.

- Enjoy!

Soba Noodle Salad

Ingredients

- ☐7 oz dried soba noodles (buckwheat noodles) (2-3 bundles for 4 servings)

- ☐2 green onions/scallions

- ☐1 handful cilantro (coriander) (0.7 oz, 20 g for 4 servings)

- ☐1 Tbsp toasted white sesame seeds

For the Dressing

- ☐1 Tbsp neutral-flavored oil (vegetable, rice bran, canola, etc.)

- ☐3 Tbsp roasted sesame oil

- ☐½ tsp crushed red pepper (red pepper flakes)

- ☐3 Tbsp honey (use maple syrup for vegan)

- ☐3 Tbsp soy sauce

Instructions

1. Gather all the ingredients.

2. To make the dressing, combine the vegetable oil, sesame oil, and crushed red peppers in a small saucepan.

3. Whisk it all together and infuse the oil over medium heat for 3 minutes. Alternatively, you can put these ingredients in a small microwave-safe bowl and microwave for 3 minutes. Set aside to let it cool a bit; be careful while handling as it'll get very hot.

4. Add the honey and soy sauce to the oil mixture.

5. Whisk it all together until the honey has completely dissolved.

6. Bring water to a boil in a large pot (you do not need to salt the water for cooking soba). Cook the soba noodles

according to the package instructions, but make sure they are al dente. Drain into a colander and rinse the soba noodles under cold running water. This step is important to remove the excess starch from the noodles and to stop the cooking. Drain well and transfer to a large bowl.

7. Thinly slice the green onions and chop the cilantro into small pieces.

8. Add the dressing, green onions, cilantro, and sesame seeds to the bowl with the soba noodles.

9. Toss everything together. Transfer to a serving bowl or plate. Serve chilled or at room temperature.

Sweet Potato Fries

INGREDIENTS

• 4 sweet potatoes, cut into large French fries

• 1 tablespoon water

• 2 teaspoons Italian seasoning

• 1/2 teaspoon lemon pepper

• 1 pinch salt and pepper to taste

• 2 tablespoons olive oil

DIRECTIONS

• Preheat the oven to 400 degrees F (200 degrees C).

• Place the cut sweet potatoes into a microwave-safe dish with the water. Cook in the microwave for 5 minutes on full power. Drain off liquid, and toss with Italian seasoning, lemon pepper, salt, pepper, and olive oil. Arrange the fries on a baking sheet in a single layer.

• Bake for 30 minutes, turning once, or until fries are crispy on the outside.

Vegan Creamy Tomato Risotto

Ingredients

Tomato Risotto:

• 1 onion

• 2 cloves of garlic

• 2 tbsp vegan butter (or olive oil)

• 150 g risotto rice

• 80 ml vegan white wine (optional, otherwise more vegetable stock)

• 250 ml vegetable broth

• 250 ml of pureed tomatoes

- approx. 50 ml coconut milk * (see recipe notes)

- 4 dried tomatoes finely chopped (optional)

- salt

- pepper

- basil

- oregano

- 1 tsp of sugar (or other sweetener)

Topping:

- cherry tomatoes

- vegan parmesan (or nutritional yeast flakes)

Instructions

- Peel the onion and cut into small cubes. Peel and chop also the garlic cloves.

• Heat up vegan butter (or olive oil) in a wide saucepan. Fry the onions and garlic until glossy for about 2-3 minutes.

• Add risotto rice and simmer for a further 1 minute while stirring. Then deglaze with white wine and cook briefly while stirring frequently.

• Reduce the heat to medium and add some vegetable stock. Cook the risotto for about 12-15 minutes. Meanwhile, gradually add vegetable stock and pureed tomatoes and stir constantly. Finally, stir in chopped dried tomatoes and some coconut milk (or plant-based cream / milk) as desired.

• Once the rice is al dente and the risotto is creamy, season with the spices and a little sugar to taste. Halve the cherry tomatoes and stir in gently.

- Serve the risotto with vegan parmesan or nutritional yeast flakes as desired.

- Enjoy your meal!

Mexican Rice

INGREDIENTS

- 3 tablespoons vegetable oil

- 1 cup uncooked long-grain rice

- 1 teaspoon garlic salt

- 1/2 teaspoon ground cumin

- 1/4 cup chopped onion

- 1/2 cup tomato sauce

- 2 cups chicken broth

DIRECTIONS

- Place a large saucepan over medium heat and add oil. Add rice and stir constantly until puffed and golden.

Sprinkle over salt and cumin while cooking.

• Add onions and cook until tender. Mix in tomato sauce and chicken broth. Bring to a boil.

• Reduce heat to low and cover the saucepan. Let it simmer for 20 to 25 minutes.

• Fluff rice with a fork. Enjoy!

Cracker Barrel Fried Okra

INGREDIENTS

• 1 quart fresh okra

• 2 to 3 tablespoons all-purpose flour

• 1 1/2 cups yellow plain cornmeal

• 1 egg, beaten

• 1 teaspoon salt

- 1/2 teaspoon pepper

- Canola, peanut, or vegetable oil for frying

DIRECTIONS

- Rinse okra and slice into half-inch rounds. Discard caps and bottom tips.

- Place okra slices in a mixing bowl and sprinkle them with flour. Shake vigorously to ensure even coating. Strain in a wire strainer to get rid of excess flour and get a very light coating.

- Transfer back into the mixing bowl. Stir in the egg until okra slices are well-coated.

- Place cornmeal, salt, and pepper in a ziplock bag. Shake to mix.

- Add 1 cup of okra to the bag, seal, and shake until evenly coated. Transfer them into a plate. Repeat this step for the rest of the okra slices.

• In a heavy bottom pan or cast-iron skillet, pour half-inch deep of lard or oil and heat over medium-high heat until the temperature is 350 degrees Fahrenheit.

• Fry okra slices, making sure the pan is not over-crowded until golden brown. Drain excess oil by placing okra on a wire rack lined with paper towels.

SUMMARY

A dairy-free diet excludes animal milks and any products that contain them. Some people choose to go dairy-free because they have an allergy or intolerance, while others have a personal or ethical preference. Because dairy is a source of necessary nutrients like calcium, vitamin D, and protein, experts recommend making sure to incorporate other sources of those nutrients into your daily meals.

If you're considering going dairy-free, check with a healthcare provider first, particularly if you have an underlying health condition. They'll be able to discuss the risks and benefits of a dairy-free diet based on your individual situation, or refer you to a nutritionist or dietitian. Remember that there's no one-size-fits-all approach to any of the various diet options and feel encouraged to follow what works best for you and your overall health.